PTSD RECOVERY JOURNAL

PTSD RECOVERY JOURNAL

REFLECTIVE PROMPTS and EVIDENCE-BASED PRACTICES to HELP YOU HEAL and GROW

Patricia Alvarado, LPCC

callisto
publishing
an imprint of Sourcebooks

This journal belongs to:

_____

CONTENTS

INTRODUCTION

Welcome to your *PTSD Recovery Journal*! This journal presents a meaningful opportunity to learn and reflect on your experiences and to gradually and mindfully grow and heal. My name is Patricia Alvarado and I am a licensed psychotherapist based in Los Angeles, California. I have been working in the field of mental health for more than 10 years and with trauma survivors throughout my entire career. I am an EMDR (eye movement desensitization and reprocessing) therapist and provide therapeutic services within my group practice, Alvarado Therapy. What I love most about the work that I do is the realization of the day-to-day resilience that we have. Despite the difficulties endured, we are boundlessly resilient, and that brings hope. Hope is what I wish for you as well.

Journaling is a powerful tool that can help you process and reflect on where you have been and how far you have come. As you work through this journal, remember to give yourself grace. Journaling can be healing and can help you make sense of the feelings, thoughts, and sensations you have and the reasons you have them. Journaling can also help remind you of the positive coping skills (a concept we will cover) you have been using and reflect on what more you may need within your healing journey.

Within this journal, you will work with many important phrases and concepts, including post-traumatic stress disorder, or PTSD. PTSD is identified as stress that results after a trauma we experience ourselves or have witnessed or heard about. These experiences, from things like sexual or physical assault to witnessing a car accident, living through a natural disaster, or enduring military combat, then, create stressful environments because of the triggers that may arise from them.

No matter the specifics of the trauma you experienced, you may notice tension in your body or overwhelming feelings running through you when you work through each prompt and practice in this journal. Although it can feel intimidating at first, please remember that you have the option to stay on one page, take a break, or continue moving forward, but always at your own pace. Take deep breaths throughout and continuously remind yourself that you are in control at this time. You are allowed to take things slow. I am in your corner and am here to guide you through the process.

The goal of this journal is to offer you guidance and helpful tools to manage and understand your PTSD symptoms, so you feel safe and in control during your healing and recovery. Be patient with yourself. Be gentle with yourself. You are exactly where you need to be.

HOW TO USE THIS JOURNAL

As you work through each section in this journal, you will notice that each builds upon the other, establishing a greater understanding of PTSD and promoting recovery from it, helping you engage in a mindful process of healing. This journal is designed to be worked sequentially, with each section's concepts building and layering on the previous. Work your way through it gradually, at your pace, and hold compassion for yourself as you do so.

In the first section, you will begin by taking note of where you are in this specific moment in your life. In the second section, you will spend time learning about thoughts and feelings that may influence your behaviors. And in the third, you will focus on your body and the reactions you may be having to your thoughts and feelings. In the fourth and final section, you will come to understand how gradual healing occurs, remembering there are no specific time lines to it. Each section includes prompts to get you thinking and practices to put that thinking into motion. You will also encounter affirmations that create a positive and encouraging environment, providing words to turn to in moments of overwhelm or unease during your healing journey.

Flexibility is key when thinking about interacting with and using this journal. When considering the best time to work through the journal, think about your day and determine where journaling fits in. Listen to that inner voice and those subtle daily rhythms and let them guide you. You may notice that you want to work through the journal as part of your morning routine or during a specific day on the weekend.

There are no rules about when you do the work, so long as it makes sense for your life. If you create a plan that doesn't work, change it to something that feels better and meets your needs.

This journal offers great tools to help you further your PTSD healing and recovery, but by no means is it a replacement for professional services with a mental health provider. Here, we'll discuss various feelings surrounding guilt, hopelessness, sadness, and shame as well as tools to help you work through the difficulties you are experiencing. If you notice that you need additional support and guidance, please do not hesitate to reach out to a mental health professional and visit the Resources section (page 137) for further outreach suggestions. There is no shame in seeking help or treatment; the most important thing is that you feel safe and supported.

Acknowledge the great step you've made to take care of *you* by using this journal. This is a great starting point, and there is only more to learn moving forward. Healing and recovery are yours to claim.

Acknowledging Where You Are

You may have many questions and thoughts throughout this process, such as, "Will I ever feel normal again?" "No one understands what I am going through," "I feel alone in all of this." It's understandable to have these thoughts, feelings, and questions when something scary or traumatic happens, and it can feel like nothing will ever be the same. Let's reflect on that for a moment.

Although things may never be the same, that doesn't mean you will never be okay. Change is okay. Healing happens through change, and when you learn about where you are within your process, you can begin to be comfortable with the uncomfortable.

The themes within this section are intended to help you understand your experience, notice it, and normalize it, so you can begin to heal from it. You will learn to identify what PTSD is by reflecting on your experiences. You will learn what a fight-or-flight response is and practice working with effective tools that will help you stay in your body when challenging moments arise. By reflecting on past work, you will begin to notice your progress as you are guided toward continued healing.

Remember, this is your process and you can take it as fast or as slow as you need to. There is no rush. Pay attention to how you feel when working through each journal section. Make space, be patient with yourself, and, above all, be compassionate with yourself in this moment.

You may wonder, "What is trauma anyway? Have I experienced trauma? Do I have PTSD?" These are normal questions to ask as you learn more about yourself. Write down what made you choose this journal and decide that it could be helpful for you.

_____

_____

_____

_____

_____

_____

_____

_____

_____

_____

_____

_____

_____

_____

_____

_____

_____

_____

_____

_____

_____

_____

_____

PTSD is identified as stress that occurs after a trauma due to situations we experience ourselves or have witnessed or heard about. These can be life-threatening situations, community violence, or any type of abuse—emotional, physical, sexual, or neglect during childhood, adolescence, or adulthood. Trauma can present itself in many ways. As you consider this fact, what questions come up right now?

_____

_____

_____

_____

_____

_____

_____

_____

_____

_____

_____

_____

_____

_____

_____

As you work through this journal, you may remember the traumatic events you experienced. You may begin to pay attention to how you felt in those difficult moments. This is common because you may be accustomed to compartmentalizing thoughts and feelings, or sweeping them "under the rug." By picking up this journal, you may feel "found out" or vulnerable as you recognize that what you have been through has resulted in PTSD. Writing about this, but more specifically writing about this to your future self, can help you acknowledge where you are right now—and see where you may find yourself in the future.

Using a separate sheet of paper, take a few moments to write a letter to your healed future self. What do you want your future self to know? What guidance can you share? How do you want your future self to feel by the end of this journal? Once the letter is finished, turn the page, and continue working through the journal at a pace that feels comfortable to you. Keep your future self in your mind and in your focus, holding that healed self with compassion as you progress through the entries and sections ahead.

As you pick up this journal and recognize what you want to work through—*trauma*—various thoughts may come up. Trauma work is difficult, and taking it one step at a time will help guide your process. Jot down any thoughts you notice in this moment.

_____

_____

_____

_____

_____

_____

_____

_____

_____

_____

_____

_____

_____

_____

_____

_____

_____

_____

_____

_____

_____

Trauma work is challenging, and understanding where you are in this moment is helpful to beginning the process. This may be the first time you have decided to work through your trauma, and that is okay. Acknowledge your feelings in this moment. How do you feel right now?

_____

_____

_____

_____

_____

_____

_____

_____

_____

_____

_____

_____

_____

_____

_____

_____

_____

_____

_____

_____

Today is the beginning of my healing journey and I honor this moment to the best of my ability. Starting now is the perfect time.

When you find yourself upset in certain situations, your anger or discomfort may be happening because you are responding to a "trigger." A trigger is something that reminds us of upsetting past events. Although the situation may not be directly linked to the past trauma, something about the situation brings it to mind and causes a reaction. When do you notice that you are triggered?

_____

_____

_____

_____

_____

_____

_____

_____

_____

_____

_____

_____

_____

_____

_____

_____

_____

_____

Creating a "coping toolbox" to help you manage PTSD can prove a means of support when you experience increased PTSD symptoms. In such moments of heightened intensity, you may notice anger, fear, guilt, sadness, or shame. Coping skills, such as deep breathing, listening to your favorite music, talking to a friend, or quiet time, can help you regulate these emotions. Which coping skills are in your toolbox already?

_____

_____

_____

_____

_____

_____

_____

_____

_____

_____

_____

_____

_____

_____

_____

_____

_____

_____

I am allowed to find calmness and peace in everything I do. I can notice how I feel as I take care of myself at this moment. I am okay as I am.

Identifying your triggers will help you manage them effectively. Recognizing what you are feeling makes that feeling easier to manage. When you can manage feelings in a more productive way, you can begin to feel better. The goal is to help prepare you for situations in which you may feel triggered. From the list that follows, check off those things that trigger you most and write in any that aren't listed here on the blank lines below.

- ☐ Returning to where my trauma occurred
- ☐ Loud noises
- ☐ Specific scents
- ☐ Certain objects
- ☐ Watching the news
- ☐ Seeing people suffer
- ☐ Insomnia
- ☐ Doctors' offices
- ☐ Driving
- ☐ Watching war movies
- ☐ Seeing certain people
- ☐ Anniversary of the event

- ☐ Loss of a loved one
- ☐ The end of a relationship
- ☐ Small spaces
- ☐ Large spaces
- ☐ Small gatherings
- ☐ Large gatherings
- ☐ Specific friends or family members
- ☐ Feeling alone or left out
- ☐ Feeling overwhelmed
- ☐ _____
- ☐ _____
- ☐ _____

Are there any patterns you notice about the triggers you checked off?

_____

_____

_____

_____

_____

_____

_____

_____

_____

_____

_____

_____

_____

_____

_____

_____

_____

During times of increased stress, you may notice that you experience a need to fight. The anger that you may feel is a common trauma response in moments of distress. Do you feel like fighting after being triggered? If so, when was the last time you felt this way?

_____

_____

_____

_____

_____

_____

_____

_____

_____

_____

_____

_____

_____

_____

_____

_____

_____

_____

_____

_____

As with the need to fight, you may alternately notice a feeling of freezing, or tensing up, in uncomfortable situations. In the moment of trauma, it may have felt scary or difficult to do anything but freeze—this is another normal response to distress. Do you feel like freezing in stressful situations? If so, when does this happen most?

_____

_____

_____

_____

_____

_____

_____

_____

_____

_____

_____

_____

_____

_____

_____

_____

_____

_____

_____

_____

Fleeing or running away from uncomfortable thoughts, feelings, or situations is a defense mechanism you may have developed to help you cope with negative emotions. Again, this is normal behavior even if it doesn't *seem* normal. What situations cause you to choose avoidance and make you want to flee?

_____

_____

_____

_____

_____

_____

_____

_____

_____

_____

_____

_____

_____

_____

_____

_____

_____

_____

_____

Being aware of the common reactions you have when you feel threatened or triggered can cause you to experience intense emotions, such as fear, increased sadness, or low motivation. What do you do when you feel this way? What other intense emotions do you struggle with at this time?

_____

_____

_____

_____

_____

_____

_____

_____

_____

_____

_____

_____

_____

_____

_____

_____

_____

_____

_____

_____

_____

When making the decision to begin healing, you may also have questions about why this trauma happened to you. You may feel hopeless and undeserving because of the experiences you went through. Remember, PTSD is a result of the loss of power you experienced during your trauma. Allow yourself to question, with compassion and curiosity, to help you understand that how you feel today is normal, given your experiences. Whether your trauma occurred during your childhood, as a teenager, or during adulthood, your feelings are valid because they are unique to you. Allow yourself time and be patient with yourself as you reflect on the following questions:

- How old do I feel as I begin working through this journal?

- What is the hardest part about what I feel right now?

- What is something I am proud of right now?

- What kind of commitment can I make to help myself complete this journal?

Keep these answers in mind as you progress through your healing journey.

The mind is powerful. It can dictate how we feel, react, and respond to people or events throughout the day. Trauma alters the way we think about things because of the experiences we have had, and you may have subconsciously created defenses to help you cope with them. What kinds of things do you do to defend yourself?

_____

_____

_____

_____

_____

_____

_____

_____

_____

_____

_____

_____

_____

_____

_____

_____

_____

_____

_____

When we have intense emotions, our minds may "spiral." Spiraling begins when you have one negative thought, then another, and another, and suddenly you are plummeting down a rabbit hole of negative thoughts. It can feel hard to stop your thoughts from going into a spiral. Write down the people, places, or things that may cause you to spiral.

_____

_____

_____

_____

_____

_____

_____

_____

_____

_____

_____

_____

_____

_____

_____

_____

_____

_____

_____

_____

_____

I continuously learn about myself, even when some parts of me are harder to manage than others. I am still learning about these parts and trying to be as present as possible.

Hypervigilance, or increased alertness, occurs when our sympathetic nervous system begins to prepare for action. (To learn more about the sympathetic nervous system, see page 78.) In such moments, you may find yourself noticing everything around you and feeling as though you are in danger. Although the danger may not be real, your past trauma may make it feel very real. What kinds of situations cause you to be hypervigilant?

_____

_____

_____

_____

_____

_____

_____

_____

_____

_____

_____

_____

_____

_____

_____

_____

_____

_____

Your body responds to the thoughts you are thinking in a way that can feel profoundly physical. You may notice aches and pains, difficulty breathing, indigestion, or insomnia, among other things. These are called "psychosomatic symptoms" and they are caused when you are flooded with emotions. How does your body respond during moments of intense emotions?

_____

_____

_____

_____

_____

_____

_____

_____

_____

_____

_____

_____

_____

_____

_____

_____

_____

_____

_____

Noticing your breath will help you calm your nervous system and recognize that you are okay in this moment. The trauma that you experienced is *not* happening in this instant, even if it feels as though you are reliving past events. Breathing is something we do consciously and unconsciously. Sometimes you may notice that you are breathing heavily while other times you may notice you are breathing shallowly or holding your breath. Breathing with intention can help you decrease any stress you may be holding, increase calm, and help you feel clearer. Try this easy and effective breathing technique you can begin using today:

1. Sit comfortably and close your eyes, or gaze down resting one hand on your chest and the other hand softly on your belly.

2. Begin noticing the natural rhythm of your breath.

3. Slowly inhale through your nose for four seconds and softly exhale through your mouth for four seconds.

4. Repeat this exercise three times, or as many times as you need.

When you know there are others who relate to what you have been through, you may begin to feel like you are not alone. This is what we call "normalizing" experiences. Normalizing can happen in various situations and can be especially helpful as you work through your trauma. It can be reassuring to know that others have experienced something similar to you. As you explore your feelings and emotions, what kind of things can you tell yourself to help normalize your experiences?

_____

_____

_____

_____

_____

_____

_____

_____

_____

_____

_____

_____

_____

_____

_____

_____

_____

When it comes to your personal trauma and reflecting on your experience, you may feel that it will be difficult or scary to complete this journal and uncover your emotions and feelings about your unique life events. Take breaks throughout the process and always do what feels comfortable. Know that healing takes time. What are some go-to activities you can engage in if journaling becomes too overwhelming? Jot them down here.

_____

_____

_____

_____

_____

_____

_____

_____

_____

_____

_____

_____

_____

_____

_____

_____

*I am worthy of compassion. I am capable
of experiencing happiness and joy.
I will feel good today and tomorrow despite
what I have been through in my life.*

Although it can feel as though you are experiencing too many emotions all the time, remember that emotions change based on the situation and moment by moment. Be compassionate with yourself as you continue learning about yourself, your trauma, and your reactions to your trauma. What are three things you can do to show yourself extra kindness or compassion?

_____

_____

_____

_____

_____

_____

_____

_____

_____

_____

_____

_____

_____

_____

_____

_____

_____

_____

Taking loving care of yourself throughout this journaling process will allow you to go deeper with your healing work. As you continue to normalize your experiences, you will slowly feel the work presented in this journal becoming easier to move through. What acts of self-care do you practice already? What would you like to add to the list? Writing them here will remind you later, when you need to take a moment for yourself.

We all need someone to rely on, like a trusted family member, friend, or mentor. As you think about this fact, remind yourself of times you needed help in other areas of your life. Did you need help bagging groceries, changing a tire, or learning a new task at work?

Having supportive people to lean on can help you manage your feelings in moments of distress. This does not necessarily mean these people need to know what you went through. It simply means they can be a sounding board when needed, or offer help if you ask for it. Take a few moments to think about someone you feel comfortable reaching out to when you have a bad day. Consider the following questions to guide your reflections:

- What is it about this person that you enjoy?

- What kind of help can you imagine asking for?

- Has this person been supportive of you in the past?

- How much are you willing to share?

Refer to this page when you are having a difficult day and want to ask for help. This exercise will remind you of the reasons you identified this support person in the first place.

Approach yourself with the utmost compassion. Compassion allows you to accept and respect yourself, be okay with how you feel, and helps you to recognize your strengths. Although compassion may feel impossible today, remember that over time, it may come more easily. You are slowly healing. How often do you show yourself compassion? How can you allow yourself compassion as you continue learning about PTSD?

_____

_____

_____

_____

_____

_____

_____

_____

_____

_____

_____

_____

_____

_____

_____

_____

_____

_____

Understand the power you have. Often, PTSD comes from feeling powerless. Something terrible happened that took away or muted your power. Now, it's time to take back your power. Imagine how it can feel to be full of power and control. What does that look like for you?

_____

_____

_____

_____

_____

_____

_____

_____

_____

_____

_____

_____

_____

_____

_____

_____

_____

_____

_____

Even though I acknowledge that I have felt powerless in the past, I recognize that I am powerful today. What I have gone through has only made me stronger.

SECTION TWO

Thoughts, Feelings, and Behaviors

By now, you are beginning to understand what trauma is and how your experiences play a role in how you feel throughout the day. You're starting to understand what PTSD is, and you may be asking yourself, "Why do I still feel this way?"

In this section, we will explore how our thoughts affect our feelings and, in turn, how our feelings affect our behaviors. As you continue on the path toward healing, you will begin to understand the common symptoms affecting many people with PTSD. Although it can seem like you are the only one feeling this way, you are not alone.

When trauma is ignored, it can show up in unexpected ways. You may have trouble sleeping or experience nightmares or feel jumpy in situations where you once felt at ease. You may also notice frustrated, irritated, or moody feelings at times when these reactions do not make sense, but for some reason they are hard to shake. People, places, or things can cause you to think continuously about the traumatic experience you endured. Feelings of disappointment, guilt, sadness, or shame may cause you to feel helpless and hopeless.

These reactions are caused by intrusive thoughts surrounding your trauma. We will explore why this happens and what may be helpful for your recovery.

Because our thoughts are so powerful, they can create both good and bad feelings. Feelings, then, affect the way we react to situations. If you have a negative thought, chances are you will have a negative feeling. What do you notice about the relationship between your thoughts and your feelings?

_____

_____

_____

_____

_____

_____

_____

_____

_____

_____

_____

_____

_____

_____

_____

_____

_____

_____

_____

_____

_____

When thoughts affect feelings, feelings then influence the way we behave in situations. If you have an unhelpful thought, an unhelpful feeling may be triggered that will cause an unhelpful reaction. What are the common reactions you have when you experience a bad thought and feeling?

_____

_____

_____

_____

_____

_____

_____

_____

_____

_____

_____

_____

_____

_____

_____

_____

_____

_____

_____

_____

_____

Noticing your thoughts is a helpful way to understand the feelings you experience and, with that, the actions you take as a result of those feelings. If you can notice specific thoughts that cause you to feel overwhelmed or stressed, you can practice "thought stopping."

Thought stopping is literally that: stopping thoughts from taking over how you feel. These thoughts may be things that cause you to doubt yourself, your experience, your abilities, or your judgment. Let's practice thought stopping:

Think of the last time you felt stressed or overwhelmed. What thought was present? (For example, "I am going to fail this test!" "My boss is going to be upset with me!" "I have so many things to do around the house!")

How did you feel (e.g., angry, disappointed, frustrated, sad) as a result of the thought?

What was your behavior? (For example, I am not going to participate. I am going to call in sick to work. I am going to sit here because there's too much to do.)

Do you notice how your thoughts, feelings, and behaviors all played a role in the situation? As you review your thoughts, say out loud, "STOP." What can you tell yourself instead? How does saying "STOP" change how you feel and behave thereafter?

PTSD can cause us to experience many things, including negative thought patterns. Identifying how you feel and behave in situations will help you notice the negative thought patterns that resurface, causing your rumination. How do your negative thought patterns stop you from doing the things you want to do?

_____

_____

_____

_____

_____

_____

_____

_____

_____

_____

_____

_____

_____

_____

_____

_____

_____

_____

_____

_____

_____

Rumination, or focusing intently on or reviewing things repeatedly in our mind, is what we often do when we wonder whether we did the right thing or made the right decision, and when we are consistently bargaining with ourselves about our decisions. PTSD can cause us to doubt everything we ever believed. How often do you find yourself affected by the things you ruminate over?

_____

_____

_____

_____

_____

_____

_____

_____

_____

_____

_____

_____

_____

_____

_____

_____

_____

_____

I can acknowledge thoughts, feelings, and behaviors and I have the power to change them. I can approach thoughts, feelings, and behaviors judgment-free. I have the power.

Since the trauma occurred, you may experience thoughts, feelings, or emotions that you did not experience before, such as flashbacks. Flashbacks can feel like they come out of nowhere, and you may also experience physical or emotional symptoms because of them. Just as you can have a flashback of joyful moments and successful milestones in your life, you can experience flashbacks of upsetting situations as well, feeling as though you are reliving those experiences. Describe what your flashbacks feel like. How do they manifest for you?

_____

_____

_____

_____

_____

_____

_____

_____

_____

_____

_____

_____

_____

_____

_____

_____

_____

_____

Each of us develops defense mechanisms that protect us in moments of crisis. Defense mechanisms are things like denial or blocking memories and can vary depending on the setting. These defense mechanisms are also considered trauma responses. What are the defense mechanisms you use to protect yourself? How comfortable do you feel when using them—and afterward?

_____

_____

_____

_____

_____

_____

_____

_____

_____

_____

_____

_____

_____

_____

_____

_____

_____

_____

How you feel about yourself affects the way you approach things in your daily life, and journaling can help you sort out those feelings.

Stream-of-consciousness journaling is a great tool anyone can use, and it can be done in whatever way makes the most sense for you. Journaling may feel like something you cannot connect to, but once you try it, you may notice that this different approach can be helpful in processing thoughts and feelings. Remember, thoughts, feelings, and behaviors are intertwined.

Using thought stopping to decrease self-defeating thoughts, pull out a sheet of paper and write about how you have felt this week. Write about anything: how you felt in a specific situation, how you feel about another person, or how you feel overall.

If judgment presents itself, say "STOP" and keep going. While journaling, feel free to use bullet points, words, phrases, and complete or incomplete sentences. Stream of consciousness is encouraged.

When you are done, fold the sheet of paper and put it in a safe place. If you are writing in a notebook, fold the page and close the notebook. You don't have to reread what you wrote unless you want to.

Every experience is unique, and what you feel right now is significant because it's happening to you. There is no right or wrong feeling to have in a given moment, as growth happens when we are self-aware. Briefly describe one or two times when you didn't give your feelings enough value. Know that accepting where you are in your process is the first step.

_____

_____

_____

_____

_____

_____

_____

_____

_____

_____

_____

_____

_____

_____

_____

_____

_____

_____

_____

Even though something very difficult happened to you, you can still experience positive feelings. Although those good feelings may be harder to come by nowadays, can you think about a recent occasion when you felt content, excited, happy, or hopeful? This could be any occasion. Small wins count, too.

_____

_____

_____

_____

_____

_____

_____

_____

_____

_____

_____

_____

_____

_____

_____

_____

_____

_____

_____

_____

Even though things can be scary or uncomfortable,
I can acknowledge moments when I am okay.
I am capable of healing. I deserve healing.

You may expect something bad to happen, causing you to experience uncomfortable feelings. The thoughts you have may even cause you to approach situations with the idea that nothing will go right. Remember, our thoughts are very powerful. What kind of bad things do you always expect to happen? Now, consider the likelihood that these bad things will actually happen. What do you notice?

_____

_____

_____

_____

_____

_____

_____

_____

_____

_____

_____

_____

_____

_____

_____

_____

_____

_____

Thought distortions are negative thoughts we have about ourselves or situations that may not actually be true. You may notice thought distortions when you are unclear in certain situations or you begin to doubt yourself and your decisions. These distortions can be things like quickly jumping to conclusions or not acknowledging when things go well. What kind of thought distortions do you typically have?

_____

_____

_____

_____

_____

_____

_____

_____

_____

_____

_____

_____

_____

_____

_____

_____

_____

How often do you ask someone how they feel and they respond, "Good"? Let's remember, good is not a feeling! Although this is a common response, it's a superficial response that does not create space for vulnerability. The differences between thoughts and feelings can be confusing, but with time and practice, you can master their recognition. Doing so will also help you identify strong boundaries (we will explore more on boundaries on page 130), so you can be comfortable when sharing.

Following is a list of common thoughts and feelings. Please check off the ones that are **feelings**:

- ☐ Sometimes when I am upset, I feel as if I can't do anything right.

- ☐ When we spend time together, I feel excited about the things we will accomplish.

- ☐ I feel hopeful about the future.

- ☐ I need to take a deep breath.

- ☐ I feel lonely.

- ☐ I am feeling good today.

How did you do? Check the answer key below to gauge how your responses align. How often do you use thoughts instead of feelings to avoid deeper conversations?

Answers: thought, feeling, feeling, thought, feeling, thought

The situations we find ourselves in throughout our day, either in person, through watching television, or while interacting on social media, can trigger us. At times, we may not realize we have been triggered, but we might notice uncomfortable thoughts and feelings. Think about the last time you were uncomfortable; what was the situation?

_____

_____

_____

_____

_____

_____

_____

_____

_____

_____

_____

_____

_____

_____

_____

_____

_____

Understanding what triggers your PTSD symptoms and recognizing when you experience them will help you find ways to self-soothe. Self-soothing is a comforting way to calm yourself in times of distress. You cannot predict every situation that will trigger you, but understanding a few possibilities will shed light on what causes you the most distress. What people, places, things, and/or sounds trigger you?

_____

_____

_____

_____

_____

_____

_____

_____

_____

_____

_____

_____

_____

_____

_____

_____

_____

_____

I am capable of changing how I feel in situations even when I feel uncomfortable. I am capable of doing things I once thought I could never do again.

You may notice reactions in your body that you did not feel before, such as anger, fear, or sadness. These feelings may be triggered during specific activities, near given places, or around certain people. These reactions may cause you to avoid these situations because the feelings may be unmanageable. What are the people, places, or things you find yourself avoiding?

_____

_____

_____

_____

_____

_____

_____

_____

_____

_____

_____

_____

_____

_____

_____

_____

_____

_____

Avoidance can occur in many ways. Besides avoiding physical people, places, or things, you may notice you avoid talking about your traumatic experience, causing you to feel distracted or confused. It's common to not want to talk about what happened. Ponder this for a moment. Do you avoid talking about your trauma? What are your reasons for wanting or not wanting to share?

_____

_____

_____

_____

_____

_____

_____

_____

_____

_____

_____

_____

_____

_____

_____

_____

_____

_____

_____

Avoidance is a common trauma response because, let's face it, if something is scary or uncomfortable, we do not want any part of it. That is a normal feeling. What is hard about avoidance is that, after a trauma, you may notice you avoid a lot of things you once felt comfortable doing. Common things that you may avoid can include specific places, certain events, or interactions with specific people.

It is helpful to imagine this situation—and your reaction in this situation. To do so, grab a separate sheet of paper and think about a situation that is simply frustrating or annoying.

On a scale of 0 to 10, where 0 is low frustration and 10 is high, rate this disturbance between 2 and 3. Now, on your paper, write down each aspect of this event; remember to keep this situation between 2 and 3 on the disturbance scale to avoid overloading yourself.

Now that you have written this down, what is it about this situation that causes you to avoid it? Go back to your coping skills on page 10 to help you self-soothe throughout this exercise.

Learning is part of our everyday life, but unlearning is something that is rarely talked about. Unlearning is the concept of acknowledging what you learned and unlearning it by doing something different. If you have learned to avoid something, try leaning into the discomfort instead and seeing how that feels. What do you notice in your body at this time of discomfort? Do you notice your heart beating a little faster or your palms getting sweaty?

_____

_____

_____

_____

_____

_____

_____

_____

_____

_____

_____

_____

_____

_____

_____

_____

_____

_____

You may notice that you have begun to develop behaviors you were not doing before. Low motivation or procrastination may be present as well as constantly criticizing yourself. These self-defeating behaviors are developed during high-stress situations and are responses to trauma. What are your self-defeating behaviors? How do they manifest for you?

_____

_____

_____

_____

_____

_____

_____

_____

_____

_____

_____

_____

_____

_____

_____

_____

_____

_____

If today is not a good day, I can give myself grace to work on myself, to feel better tomorrow. Today's decisions will not dictate how I make decisions tomorrow. I am allowed to make mistakes.

Emotional flooding is caused by intense and overwhelming emotions. Emotional flooding happens when we are confused and feel the urge to fight, freeze, or flee. Common symptoms include crying, the inability to calm yourself down, and shortness of breath. Look back to page 10 and remind yourself of the coping skills you can use when feeling emotionally flooded. How might you use those coping skills and in what triggering situations would they come in handy?

_____

_____

_____

_____

_____

_____

_____

_____

_____

_____

_____

_____

_____

_____

_____

_____

Lately, have you felt angered easily? Do you have trouble sleeping or find it difficult to concentrate? If so, you may be experiencing hyperarousal, which is a result of overwhelming feelings due to PTSD symptoms. Hyperarousal occurs after a traumatic event and can develop over time, causing you to feel on edge, confused, and irritated, among other things. Are you currently experiencing hyper-arousal? If so, what does that look or feel like?

_____

_____

_____

_____

_____

_____

_____

_____

_____

_____

_____

_____

_____

_____

_____

_____

Hypervigilance can be exhausting because you are constantly on high alert and likely feel as though everything is a threat. As a result, you may be experiencing restlessness or increased irritability, causing you to have low patience in situations you were able to manage easily in the past. Finding ways to pause and increase rest can help you approach things differently, allowing you to process thoughts and feelings before reacting.

To do this, we will practice mindfulness to help you calm your thoughts. Review a few of the affirmations included within this section (like on pages 42, 48, and 54), and pick the one that you connect with most in this moment.

Now, sit or lie in a comfortable position. Slowly inhale for four seconds, keeping the chosen affirmation in mind. As you exhale for four seconds, keep thinking about this affirmation to allow your body to rest from hypervigilance and create space for the affirmation. Repeat three times, or as needed.

The goal of this practice is to create space for other thoughts. Remember, thoughts, feelings, and behaviors all work together. If you have different thoughts, the hope is you will feel and behave differently, too.

PTSD changes how we view things, and that may mean you feel as though you are hypervigilant at all times. Hypervigilance is triggered by trauma. You may find that you look over your shoulder constantly or feel threatened constantly. Describe the situations in which you are hypervigilant. Now go back to page 37 and review how thoughts, feelings, and behaviors play a large part in this.

_____

_____

_____

_____

_____

_____

_____

_____

_____

_____

_____

_____

_____

_____

_____

_____

_____

_____

Think of a time when you felt comfortable and content within your space. This can be anywhere and at any time in your life. As you reflect, notice what you were doing during this time. What was around you? How did you feel? Note those details here. Come back to this page when self-defeating behaviors come up, to remind yourself of a comforting time.

_____

_____

_____

_____

_____

_____

_____

_____

_____

_____

_____

_____

_____

_____

_____

_____

_____

_____

_____

_____

I am at ease with myself as I continue learning about myself today. I find comfort and wisdom in my own healing.

Focusing on Your Body

In this section, you will explore and cultivate ways you can take care of yourself, free of self-judgment.

Taking care of yourself physically and emotionally may be something that feels unnatural to you. Depending on your family background or the messages imprinted upon you throughout your life, self-care may not be a priority. You may also find that because of your PTSD symptoms, self-care has gone out the window because the focus has been simply surviving each day. Wherever you find yourself within your PTSD recovery journey, it is important to notice and understand how you feel to help you self-soothe. Remember, self-care is not a luxury; it's a necessity that everyone needs, even more so when experiencing trauma.

We will look at ways you can prioritize self-care through understanding its importance to your recovery process. You will have the opportunity to explore small things in a mindful way that can have a huge positive effect on how you feel. By paying attention to how your body responds in various situations, you will learn new tools or rediscover others to help you in moments of distress. You will begin to assess how you feel and practice healthy coping techniques that can be incorporated easily into your everyday life.

Collectively, this process will help you acknowledge the difficulties you have gone through and help you continue to show compassion for yourself in a mindful way.

Everyone's definition of self-care is different. For some, it can include a soothing bath or some reflective writing whereas for others, it includes alone time. What is your definition of self-care?

_____

_____

_____

_____

_____

_____

_____

_____

_____

_____

_____

_____

_____

_____

_____

_____

_____

_____

_____

_____

_____

It's helpful to notice where you are in this moment to see what more you may need. Reflecting on your current self-care practice, list the things you do now to take care of yourself, such as going for a walk, mindfully stretching, or doing another beneficial favorite self-care practice, and consider why they are helpful for you.

_____

_____

_____

_____

_____

_____

_____

_____

_____

_____

_____

_____

_____

_____

_____

_____

_____

_____

_____

Scanning your body can help you notice any tension or pressure you may be holding in it, without judging yourself for holding it. By paying attention to this pressure or tension, you can be much more mindful of the emotional or environmental factors that trigger you. To perform a body scan:

- Begin by sitting or lying in a comfortable position. Close your eyes, or gaze down softly and pay attention to your natural breath. Notice how you are breathing, in and out.

- Redirect your focus to how your face feels, paying special attention to your jaw, tongue, and eyes. Are you clenching your jaw?

- Continue moving your focus to how your throat, shoulders, and back feel while breathing softly into these spaces.

- Then, notice how your arms, hands, and fingers feel. It may feel good to clench your hands and release the tension.

- Continue moving through your body, noticing your stomach, calves, and feet.

- Finally, move through your entire body at once and notice where you are holding any tension or pressure while you continue breathing.

Gently open your eyes. Take a sheet of paper and write down where you feel tension in your body.

Noticing where you hold stress within your body will help you further identify how you feel in this exact moment. Do you notice that you are clenching your jaw or your fingers or toes? Are you unconsciously tightening any muscles in your body? Are you experiencing headaches or stomachaches? Write down where you notice stress within your body at this moment.

_____

_____

_____

_____

_____

_____

_____

_____

_____

_____

_____

_____

_____

_____

_____

_____

_____

_____

You know that trauma affects you emotionally, but did you know that trauma also affects how you feel physically? Our brain is the "control center," and when you are triggered, the brain sends signals of discomfort, manifesting in common reactions such as cold sweat or jitters. What physical sensations do you experience when triggered?

_____

_____

_____

_____

_____

_____

_____

_____

_____

_____

_____

_____

_____

_____

_____

_____

_____

_____

_____

_____

_____

_____

I allow myself to create calm and peace within me. I am allowed to create space for myself and feel hopeful.

After you have been through a traumatic event, you may find that you stop doing the things that you used to do in the past, not only in various triggering situations but also more broadly in how you take care of yourself. Take a moment to identify self-care practices you enjoyed in the past but no longer do.

_____

_____

_____

_____

_____

_____

_____

_____

_____

_____

_____

_____

_____

_____

_____

_____

_____

_____

_____

_____

_____

Understanding the parts of the nervous system will help you understand how your body reacts to trauma. When you experience intense feelings within your body, the sympathetic nervous system prepares for action. Telltale signs include an elevated heart rate, heavy breathing, high blood pressure, and sweating. What environmental factors cause you to shift into this state?

_____

_____

_____

_____

_____

_____

_____

_____

_____

_____

_____

_____

_____

_____

_____

_____

_____

_____

_____

Adding a calm, peaceful place to your toolbox of self-soothing activities can help you create space within, where you can seek refuge when uncomfortable feelings arise.

Let's put this into practice: Think of a place that brings you calm and peace. Remember, this is a place where you can find tranquility, whether it's somewhere you have been or an imaginary place. Next, close your eyes and imagine yourself in this place, thinking about what you notice around you. Gently ask yourself these questions and take note of what you observe.

- What do you see?

- What scents do you notice?

- What sounds do you notice?

- What, if anything, can you taste?

- What can you touch?

- Where are you within this place?

Softly open your eyes. On a separate sheet of paper, write down the things you noticed that gave life to this calm, peaceful place. Completing this exercise will allow you to recognize and access this place easily when discomfort arises.

Within the nervous system, we also have a parasympathetic nervous system, which controls the body, especially while at rest, including lowering our blood pressure, breathing rate, and heart rate. What kind of environmental factors (people, surroundings, and situations) help you shift into this relaxed state?

_____

_____

_____

_____

_____

_____

_____

_____

_____

_____

_____

_____

_____

_____

_____

_____

_____

_____

_____

Although we know that sleep is important to overall functioning, it is especially significant when experiencing PTSD symptoms. Proper sleep allows your body to rest fully and to be more alert during waking hours. This allows you to approach triggers from a more balanced state of mind. What do you notice about your sleep at this time? Are you losing sleep or is your sleep restless? Do you feel rested when you wake each morning?

_____

_____

_____

_____

_____

_____

_____

_____

_____

_____

_____

_____

_____

_____

_____

_____

_____

_____

Routines do not have to work against me.
I am my own authority and can be flexible with
my time as needed. Routines can help me stay
on track to help me heal.

Healthy eating is a positive way to incorporate self-care into your daily life. Being mindful of your food choices can help with your overall mood, help you focus better, and potentially decrease anxiety, depression, and stress. Thinking back to your most recent meals and your eating patterns in general, how do your eating habits affect how you feel throughout the day?

_____

_____

_____

_____

_____

_____

_____

_____

_____

_____

_____

_____

_____

_____

_____

_____

_____

_____

_____

Self-care through exercise can help reduce PTSD symptoms, as exercise can calm your nervous system while decreasing adrenaline. During exercise, the body releases endorphins that help elevate mood. How do you feel after you exercise? Remember, exercising can come in many forms, such as walking or dancing, as long as body movement is involved.

_____

_____

_____

_____

_____

_____

_____

_____

_____

_____

_____

_____

_____

_____

_____

_____

_____

_____

_____

Tapping is a practice that can help decrease anxiety and stress while you work to heal from trauma. Alternating the tapping from left to right is similar to drumming and creates bilateral stimulation.

Bilateral stimulation activates both the right and left sides of your brain to help you self-soothe. Tapping creates a calming environment in your body while helping you stay grounded and present.

Close your eyes, or gaze down. Using your hands, gently tap on your legs or knees, alternating left and right. Maintain a slow rhythm as you do this exercise and keep breathing throughout. Do this exercise between 5 and 10 times, or as many times as needed.

How did this feel? What did you prefer, legs or knees?

Now, cross your arms over your chest and tap on your shoulders, alternating left and right, keeping a slow rhythm as you continue to breathe.

How did shoulder tapping feel? Which area, shoulders or legs, felt more soothing?

Review the affirmations presented within this section. Choose one and say it to yourself as you continue tapping for 30 seconds, or longer if needed.

Creating a routine can help you plan your day in a mindful way. Start by thinking about a waking time and sleeping time that are consistent with your life. This helps your body understand when the day starts and when it ends. What other routines can you incorporate into your day? Can you add an eating schedule or exercise schedule?

_____

_____

_____

_____

_____

_____

_____

_____

_____

_____

_____

_____

_____

_____

_____

_____

_____

_____

_____

_____

It is normal to stop doing the things that used to bring you joy because your PTSD symptoms have taken the front seat. Take a moment to make a list of all the things that bring you joy and make you feel happy. This can range from spending time with your pet to reading your favorite genre of books to watching your favorite TV shows.

_____

_____

_____

_____

_____

_____

_____

_____

_____

_____

_____

_____

_____

_____

_____

_____

_____

_____

I have the emotional strength to recognize the positive things within my life, even when things do not feel as positive as I would like.

Preparing for difficult moments will help you manage your mood in an effective way. When you understand what triggers you, you are more likely to respond to situations mindfully. What things can you do to help reduce your stress? These can be anything from listening to soothing music to practicing aromatherapy or deep breathing.

_____

_____

_____

_____

_____

_____

_____

_____

_____

_____

_____

_____

_____

_____

_____

_____

_____

_____

_____

_____

_____

Freewriting can decrease stress while helping you process how you feel. The process allows you to write whatever comes to mind; there is no right or wrong way to do it. Either on this page or in your journal, begin writing, dedicating five minutes to the activity. Use all the space you need to freewrite; if you can't think of anything to write, repeat the last sentence you wrote.

_____

_____

_____

_____

_____

_____

_____

_____

_____

_____

_____

_____

_____

_____

_____

_____

_____

_____

_____

_____

_____

_____

When you feel overwhelmed during the day, identifying your emotional strengths can remind you of how powerful you are. When PTSD symptoms flare, it can be difficult to remember the good things we have within our lives because negative feelings take over the focus.

Let's begin by identifying your emotional strengths, writing in any additional ones you'd like to add after this list.

- I am an empathetic person.
- I take care of my body.
- I am flexible with my time.
- I am a good listener.
- I respond to other people's needs.

- I am organized.
- I have common sense.
- I am liked by others.
- I am patient.
- I have a good sense of humor.

_____

_____

Now that you have identified your emotional strengths, what are you most proud of, and why?

How can you use this list to help you when things seem like they are not going as planned? Remind yourself of these strengths the next time you feel PTSD symptoms coming on and need this inner reassurance the most.

Allowing yourself to feel how you feel, judgment-free, can further decrease any negative feelings that are present. Saying these thoughts out loud helps you hear this judgment and challenge it at the same time. Take a moment to say out loud the thoughts that are causing you stress. Now, reflect on them here, in writing, asking yourself and answering whether what you think is actually valid and true.

_____

_____

_____

_____

_____

_____

_____

_____

_____

_____

_____

_____

_____

_____

_____

_____

_____

_____

By now, you have identified some low-stress activities that can help you be more mindful. Creating a plan to incorporate these activities into your daily life will turn them into daily habits. Take a moment to write down three to five things you can begin doing today, even incrementally, to make a difference. Look back at page 89 to remind you of what these activities are.

_____

_____

_____

_____

_____

_____

_____

_____

_____

_____

_____

_____

_____

_____

_____

_____

_____

_____

*I have the knowledge within me to pay
attention to how my body reacts in situations.
I can say no and do things that feel better for me.*

Even though you can recognize that trauma causes you increased feelings, including stress, it's helpful to recognize that important moments, such as family gatherings or birthdays, can also cause stress. Right now, your emotions may feel heightened in general. What are the important moments that cause you stress? Look back to page 10 to remember the coping skills that help.

_____

_____

_____

_____

_____

_____

_____

_____

_____

_____

_____

_____

_____

_____

_____

_____

_____

_____

Paying attention to the small things around you in a mindful way helps you stay present in this moment. Noticing what is around you as a way to remember that you are okay can bring you comfort. Look around your space right now. What small things do you notice? Keep breathing softly as you do this activity.

_____

_____

_____

_____

_____

_____

_____

_____

_____

_____

_____

_____

_____

_____

_____

_____

_____

_____

_____

_____

_____

U sing your five senses to help you stay grounded can help you feel present within your body. The five senses are sight, sound, smell, taste, and touch.

- To do this exercise, sit in a comfortable position and follow the natural rhythm of your breath.

- Now, identify five things you see around you. These things can be anything within your space.

- Name four things you hear. Pay attention to the sounds that are present.

- How about touch? What are three things you can touch? Go ahead and touch these things.

- Now, what are two things you smell?

- Lastly, what is one thing you can taste? Run your tongue over your teeth to deepen the taste.

How do you feel now that you have activated your five senses? This practice can be used whenever you need to come back into your body and can be incorporated into your daily routine.

You do not have to use all five senses each time. You are the authority; do what feels good in the moment.

Understanding how the brain and body are connected can help you recognize how trauma is triggered. Within your brain, the frontal lobe activates the way we think and plan for things, whereas the amygdala activates trauma memories and reactions within your body. To soothe the amygdala, look at your coping toolbox (see page 10) and write down one activity you want to do more frequently.

_____

_____

_____

_____

_____

_____

_____

_____

_____

_____

_____

_____

_____

_____

_____

_____

_____

_____

On a scale of 0 to 10, with 0 being not disturbed and 10 being very disturbed, how do you feel right now? Paying attention to your breath helps decrease PTSD symptoms while increasing alertness. Take a moment to inhale through your nose, hold the inhale for two seconds, then softly exhale through your mouth. Now, rate yourself again. Did your rating change? What can you describe about how you feel within your body after taking a deep breath?

_____

_____

_____

_____

_____

_____

_____

_____

_____

_____

_____

_____

_____

_____

_____

_____

Today and always I will remember to love myself first. I am important and I am allowed to express love for myself.

Healing Is a Gradual Process

Throughout this journal, you have been introduced to powerful tools with the goal that you have learned a lot about yourself along the way. Within each section, you have discovered aspects of PTSD to help you understand your trauma, to remind you that you are not alone in your experiences. Now, the focus is continued healing and growth, reminding yourself that you are worthy of happiness.

In this section, we will uncover ways that you can take care of yourself continuously as you begin to see things through a different lens—remember, what you have experienced does not define who you are. We will explore gratitude and ways you can strengthen your support systems while setting realistic goals. There will be opportunities to reflect on how far you have come and on where you wish to go.

When thinking about trauma, keep in mind there is no time line to healing PTSD. With patience and time, you will begin to feel better because you will not only understand your trauma in a different way but also notice that, despite your trauma, you can be okay. Healing is a marathon, not a sprint. With that, remember that the future is yours and the possibilities are endless.

Having a support system around you can help you as you work toward continued healing and growth. Your support system can help bolster you when you feel low and can encourage you in happy moments. Reflect on the people who are part of your inner circle. What is it about them that feels comforting to you? What type of support do they provide that soothes you?

_____

_____

_____

_____

_____

_____

_____

_____

_____

_____

_____

_____

_____

_____

_____

Your support system doesn't have to consist of people you have known for a long time. It can include people you share common interests with, folks you met through a support group, or those whom you relate to and communicate with on the internet. Who else do you consider to be part of your extended support team at this time? How can you best ask for their support when you need it?

_____

_____

_____

_____

_____

_____

_____

_____

_____

_____

_____

_____

_____

_____

_____

_____

_____

_____

_____

While you are working through your trauma, there may be moments when you find yourself in crisis. The level of crisis can vary from low to very high, depending on how it feels to you. It is normal to be triggered; after all, you are still learning a lot about what feels comfortable and what does not feel comfortable. This is why it is important to plan for what may happen, crafting a form of PTSD-specific insurance!

Let's practice by reviewing a situation that felt like a crisis in the past.

- What was the situation you experienced?

- What kind of support did you need in that moment?

- Was there anything you could have done to improve the situation?

- Keeping these things in mind, what are some effective ways to distract yourself when triggered? Who are safe people you can reach out to when you are experiencing a crisis?

- What things can help you in these moments?

- What community resources can you rely on, if needed?

Now, let's plan. Where can you keep this information so it's handy if you need it? What kind of things need to happen for you to use your crisis plan? If you think about the 0 to 10 rating from page 99, what rating will help remind you that your crisis plan is at your disposal?

Asking for help and support can feel hard to do, but when you think about it, it may be easier than it feels. For now, think about how it could be if someone were there to help you during the hard days. How would that feel and what would it change?

_____

_____

_____

_____

_____

_____

_____

_____

_____

_____

_____

_____

_____

_____

_____

_____

_____

_____

_____

_____

Now that you have identified how it may feel to ask for support, how do you feel about actually asking? Remember, your support team includes people you know or may not know but you have identified them as people who can and do show compassion and care for you. What are some ways you might request the support you need?

Everything that I need I have in this present moment. I am the owner of my path and can release my fear and doubt. I choose peace.

When thinking about gratitude, what comes to mind? At its heart, being grateful means focusing on being thankful for the things you have. It allows you to focus on appreciation and kindness. What is your definition of gratitude? How do you incorporate gratitude within your life in big or small ways?

_____

_____

_____

_____

_____

_____

_____

_____

_____

_____

_____

_____

_____

_____

_____

_____

_____

_____

_____

_____

When we do simple things, like giving thanks or acknowledging someone's efforts, we show gratitude. Showing gratitude consistently can help us feel happier throughout our day. Think about the last time you gave thanks or acknowledged someone else. What was the situation and how did it make you feel?

_____

_____

_____

_____

_____

_____

_____

_____

_____

_____

_____

_____

_____

_____

_____

_____

_____

_____

_____

_____

Bringing gratitude into our lives is not just about saying we are grateful. Rather, it is actively putting gratitude into practice, so it becomes part of who we are. Showing gratitude for what we have can change how we view ourselves and the world around us. Intentionally showing gratitude through the medium of a journal allows us to pay attention to the small things around us and helps us keep track of the positive things within our lives.

To start this practice, grab your favorite notebook or a piece of paper. Write down five things for which you are grateful at this time. These things can be anything, from waking up this morning to spending time with a loved one.

Think about someone in your life for whom you are especially grateful. This can be someone you have identified as a safe person. Share why you are grateful for this person.

These are just some ideas—feel free to think of other things for which you are grateful in your life. Remember, this journal is dedicated to expressing appreciation. For additional gratitude journal suggestions, see the Resources section (page 137).

Although you are familiar with post-traumatic stress, you may not have heard of post-traumatic growth (or PTG). PTG is a positive psychological change that occurs despite a traumatic experience. PTG recognizes the difficulty endured as well as the personal growth that can come from it. When thinking about your healing journey, how are you different now than you were when you first started this journal? What do you hope to continue doing more of after you complete this journal?

_____

_____

_____

_____

_____

_____

_____

_____

_____

_____

_____

_____

_____

_____

_____

_____

_____

_____

It is inevitable that trauma changes you. You may notice that you appreciate things in a different way or take care of yourself differently than before the trauma happened. You may need more time to do things or to think about things before making decisions. How are you different now than you were in the past?

_____

_____

_____

_____

_____

_____

_____

_____

_____

_____

_____

_____

_____

_____

_____

_____

_____

_____

_____

Past patterns no longer limit me. I am stronger each day and welcome any new emotions present within me. I accept who I am today, tomorrow, and forever.

You may have heard the term "self-compassion" thrown around but perhaps never fully understood what it is. Self-compassion can be seen as an abstract term because it's not so much something you *do* but more so how you *feel*. When you think about self-compassion, what ideas and concepts come to mind?

_____

_____

_____

_____

_____

_____

_____

_____

_____

_____

_____

_____

_____

_____

_____

_____

_____

_____

_____

_____

As defined by Kristin Neff, PhD, who has extensively researched and actively teaches on the topic, self-compassion encompasses common humanity, mindfulness, and self-kindness. It is the idea that you can be present for what you are experiencing and notice that you are not alone. We all struggle with something. What active steps can you make to welcome compassion into your life?

_____

_____

_____

_____

_____

_____

_____

_____

_____

_____

_____

_____

_____

_____

_____

_____

_____

_____

_____

_____

Practicing continued relaxation will assist your healing process. Remember, there is no time line for healing; however long it takes for you to heal is the perfect amount of time. Continuing to actively take care of yourself with relaxation techniques can help reinforce skills and allow you to feel calmer in triggering situations.

To initiate relaxation, sit or lie in a comfortable position and put on some soothing music (if that feels right for you). Begin by tightening all the muscles in your body and hold the tension for a few seconds. Now, release. How does that feel? You may feel tension leaving your body. Repeat this sequence as many times as needed.

Next, focus on specific muscles to tighten and release. Start with your hands. Tighten your hands into fists and hold for a few seconds, then release. How does this feel?

Continue doing this with other parts of your body where you notice that you are holding tension, softly breathing into those areas throughout the exercise.

Self-love begins with you, free of self-judgment or approval from anyone else. Self-love may not always come naturally. You may feel that you need to work a little harder to feel it, put in a little more effort to notice it, and constantly quiet the voices that question your worth. What are your initial thoughts about self-love? How do you experience self-love in your daily life?

_____

_____

_____

_____

_____

_____

_____

_____

_____

_____

_____

_____

_____

_____

_____

_____

_____

_____

_____

When thinking about self-love, the first thing that often comes to mind is "Be nice to yourself." Unfortunately, we tend to be the opposite: overly critical of ourselves. Would you talk to your friends the same way you talk to yourself? Jot down at least five ways you can be nicer to yourself, and return to these in those moments when you find yourself being too inwardly critical or harsh.

_____

_____

_____

_____

_____

_____

_____

_____

_____

_____

_____

_____

_____

_____

_____

_____

_____

_____

_____

_____

I can let go of all expectations around me at this time. I can feel free and powerful. I am deserving of freedom and continued light.

Before beginning this PTSD recovery journal, you may have felt as though there was no hope. Perhaps you did not want to plan for anything because it could cause upsetting feelings. What kind of things can you now plan for the next week? How about the next month?

_____

_____

_____

_____

_____

_____

_____

_____

_____

_____

_____

_____

_____

_____

_____

_____

_____

_____

_____

_____

_____

_____

Planning for the future helps motivation, aids you in organizing your goals, and instills an enduring sense of hope. With something to look forward to, we are much more likely to achieve our goals. Write down one long-term goal that you have. Take it a step further and read it out loud to bring it to life. Once you've said it aloud, return to the page and write down ways you can bring yourself one step (or several steps!) closer to achieving your goal.

_____

_____

_____

_____

_____

_____

_____

_____

_____

_____

_____

_____

_____

_____

_____

_____

_____

I am grateful for the lessons learned and the lessons to come. I receive all messages with an open heart and a willingness to learn.

Creating goals during a difficult time is especially helpful when motivation may be low or it feels like hope is lost. Knowing what we are working toward, and why, helps us stay on track in moments of challenge, overwhelm, and despair. Creating goals keeps us focused and less distracted because we have something we want to achieve.

To help set goals for a healthy future, visualize what you want to achieve and why achieving it is important to you. Look back to page 124 to remind you of what you have thought of already. Now, picture the goal in your mind and think about how it would feel to achieve it. Write it down.

- Is your goal realistic?

- What role does your goal play in your overall life?

- How long will it take to achieve this goal?

- What obstacles could get in the way of achieving your goal?

- How will you overcome these challenges?

- How will you know you have achieved your goal? What will it feel like once you have achieved it?

_____

_____

_____

_____

_____

_____

_____

_____

_____

_____

_____

_____

_____

_____

_____

_____

_____

_____

Forgiveness is an important part of the healing process. Forgiveness is not an easy task, but it can help you feel lighter, more relieved, and happier in the long term. This does not mean that you forgive what happened to you, but instead you do not allow that inner pain to guide you. Imagine how you would feel if you were able to forgive. How would you view life differently?

_____

_____

_____

_____

_____

_____

_____

_____

_____

_____

_____

_____

_____

_____

_____

_____

_____

_____

Look back at your coping skills toolbox on page 10. How has your toolbox grown with the use of this journal? What favorite coping skills do you enjoy using when intense feelings arise due to your trauma? What are some new skills, or some tried-and-true ones, that have helped your healing?

_____

_____

_____

_____

_____

_____

_____

_____

_____

_____

_____

_____

_____

_____

_____

_____

_____

_____

_____

_____

_____

Maintaining healthy personal boundaries throughout your healing journey is critical. Boundaries are limits you set and that you expect others to adhere to as they interact with you. This allows you to create positive relationships in which your physical and emotional safety is respected. Have you ever used boundaries in the past? How might boundaries help with your healing? What are some boundaries you would like to set and be firm in maintaining for yourself—and with others?

_____

_____

_____

_____

_____

_____

_____

_____

_____

_____

_____

_____

_____

_____

_____

_____

_____

_____

Protecting your peace is important as you move through your healing journey. Boundaries will play a critical role regarding who you do and don't allow into your life. There can be a physical and emotional boundary that you set with certain people to help you feel safe. With whom do you need to implement a boundary and why?

_____

_____

_____

_____

_____

_____

_____

_____

_____

_____

_____

_____

_____

_____

_____

_____

_____

_____

_____

_____

_____

Finding ways to self-regulate is important, and one way, putting things to the side, as in a container, will help you manage your emotions differently.

With a container, you can temporarily and intentionally put away thoughts and feelings that come up during inappropriate times. By doing this, you welcome mindfulness into your space and then work through triggers when you are ready and in a place to do so.

The container can be physical or imagined; for now, let's practice with a physical container. Choose something around you that, ideally, opens and closes.

Grab a piece of paper and write down any negative thoughts and feelings you notice. Fold the paper and put it into your container. Close it and put away the container.

- How did that exercise feel?

- What kind of traumatic symptoms can you imagine putting into your container?

- Now, visualize putting those traumatic thoughts and feelings into your container. How did that feel?

- Do you prefer writing things down or visualizing yourself doing this?

It is inevitable that certain places, people, smells, or sounds will trigger a negative emotion related to your trauma. This can be very upsetting. List some of those places, people, or smells that cause distress. Look back to page 129 and review the coping skills you can use in these situations. Remember, we all need support no matter where we are on our healing journey.

_____

_____

_____

_____

_____

_____

_____

_____

_____

_____

_____

_____

_____

_____

_____

_____

_____

_____

You may be familiar with the term "resilience." Resilience is the ability to recover from things that have happened to us. You may not think this term applies to you, but I encourage you to think about how far you have come. You are resilient. How does that feel? What small wins can you identify?

_____

_____

_____

_____

_____

_____

_____

_____

_____

_____

_____

_____

_____

_____

_____

_____

_____

_____

_____

_____

_____

_____

I choose to feel good today and every day.
I am capable of acknowledging opportunities and
accepting what is yet to come. I feel free.

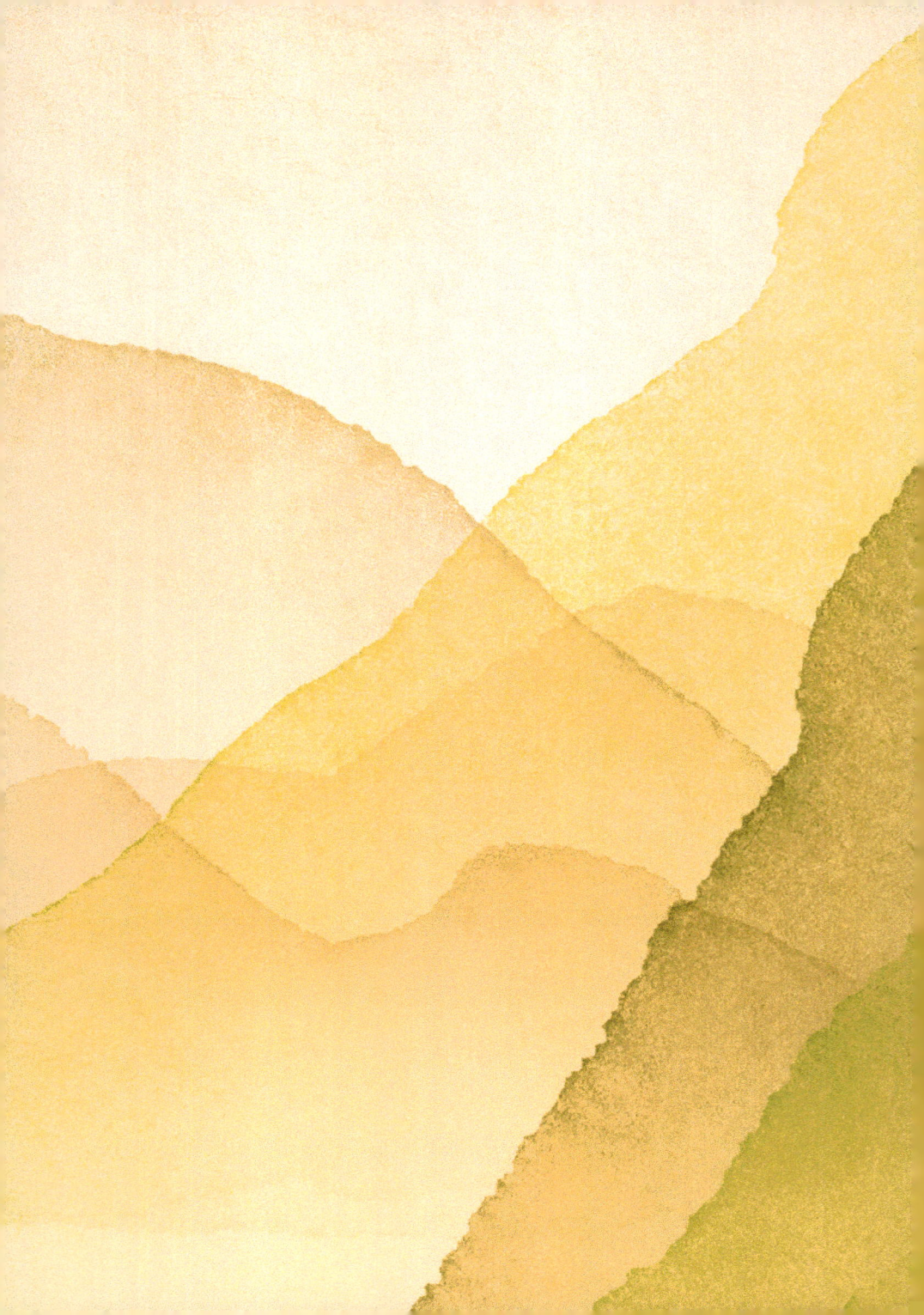

RESOURCES

From written to digital resources, there is a wealth of helpful ways to further your healing journey. Here are a few selected resources you may find especially helpful.

JOURNALS

A Year of Gratitude Journal: 52 Weeks of Prompts and Exercises to Cultivate Positivity and Joy by Keir Brady, LMFT

The 5-Minute Gratitude Journal: Give Thanks, Practice Positivity, Find Joy by Sophia Godkin, PhD

A Year of Mindfulness: A 52-Week Guided Journal to Cultivate Peace and Presence by Jennifer Raye

BOOKS

Healing PTSD: A CBT Workbook for Taking Back Your Life by Sabrina Mauro, PsyD

Practicing Mindfulness: 75 Essential Meditations to Reduce Stress, Improve Mental Health, and Find Peace in the Everyday by Matthew Sockolov

The Complex PTSD Workbook: A Mind-Body Approach to Regaining Emotional Control & Becoming Whole by Arielle Schwartz, PhD

A Year of Self-Care: Daily Practices and Inspiration for Caring for Yourself by Dr. Zoe Shaw

WEBSITES

BetterHelp: "Do I Have Post-Traumatic Stress Disorder: A PTSD Questionnaire." BetterHelp.com/advice/ptsd/do-i-have-post -traumatic-stress-disorder-a-ptsd-questionnaire

National Alliance on Mental Illness: "7 Tools for Managing Traumatic Stress." NAMI.org/Blogs/NAMI-Blog/October-2020/7-Tools-for -Managing-Traumatic-Stress

National Alliance on Mental Illness: "Posttraumatic Stress Disorder." NAMI.org/About-Mental-Illness/Mental-Health-Conditions /Posttraumatic-Stress-Disorder

National Center for PTSD: PTSD.va.gov

Psychology Today: "What Is Trauma?" PsychologyToday.com/us /basics/trauma

The National Child Traumatic Stress Network: NCTSN.org

REFERENCES

Collier, Lorna. "Growth after Trauma." *Monitor on Psychology* 47, no. 10 (2016): 48. APA.org/monitor/2016/11/growth-trauma.

Delaney, Eileen. "The Relationship between Traumatic Stress, PTSD, and Cortisol." US Naval Center for Combat and Operational Stress Control. Last modified May 2013. archive.org/details/ptsd-and-cortisol-051413.

Friedman, Matthew, Terence M. Keane, and Patricia A. Resick, eds. *Handbook of PTSD: Science and Practice*, 2nd ed. New York City: Guilford Press, 2015.

Guerry, John D., and Paul D. Hastings. "In Search of HPA Axis Dysregulation in Child and Adolescent Depression." *Clinical Child and Family Psychology Review* 14, no. 2 (June 2011): 135–160. Published online February 3, 2011.

Herman, Judith. *Trauma and Recovery: The Aftermath of Violence—From Domestic Abuse to Political Terror*, rev. ed. New York City: Basic Books, 2015.

Houston, Elaine. "What Is Goal Setting and How to Do It Well." Last modified December 28, 2020. PositivePsychology.com/goal-setting.

Kendall, Philip C., and Kristina A. Hedtke. *The Coping Cat Workbook*, 2nd ed. Ardmore, PA: Workbook Publishing, 2006.

Najavits, Lisa M. *Seeking Safety: A Model for PTSD and/or Substance Use.* New York City: Guilford Press, 2002.

Neff, Kristen. *Self-Compassion.* Self-Compassion.org.

Paulus, Martin P., and Murray B. Stein. "Interoception in Anxiety and Depression." *Brain Structure and Function* 214, nos. 5–6 (2010): 451–463. doi.org/10.1007/s00429-010-0258-9.

ACKNOWLEDGMENTS

I would like to give my warmest thanks to my closest loved ones who have been encouraging and motivating throughout this entire process. Their guidance has helped carry me throughout the writing of this journal, allowing me to reflect on experiences and understand my "why."

I would also like to give special thanks to all those raising children to the best of their ability. May we raise children who are encouraged to use their voices and notice their strengths in times of adversity. We are resilient, and we can overcome.

ABOUT THE AUTHOR

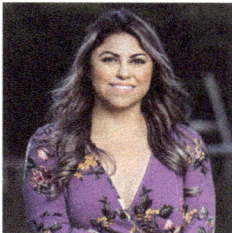

Patricia Alvarado, LPCC, is a dually licensed psychotherapist with more than 10 years of experience within the mental health field. Her experience comes from working within community mental health, volunteering on the suicide hotline, the managed care/corporate sector, and private practice. She has focused much of her work on trauma and trauma healing. Patricia is a certified EMDR therapist and owns a group practice, Alvarado Therapy, in Los Angeles, California. She hosts the *Therapy, Etc*. podcast, a biweekly conversation focusing on all things mental health. You can find Patricia sharing thoughtful and insightful messages on her Instagram accounts, @alvaradotherapy and @therapyetcpodcast.

www.ingramcontent.com/pod-product-compliance
Lightning Source LLC
Chambersburg PA
CBHW050820090426
42737CB00022B/3459